Dedicated to Conor and Margaret, who inspired this story,

and to their parents, Abby and Chrys,

whose photographs helped me create the pictures.

My Brother Came Early

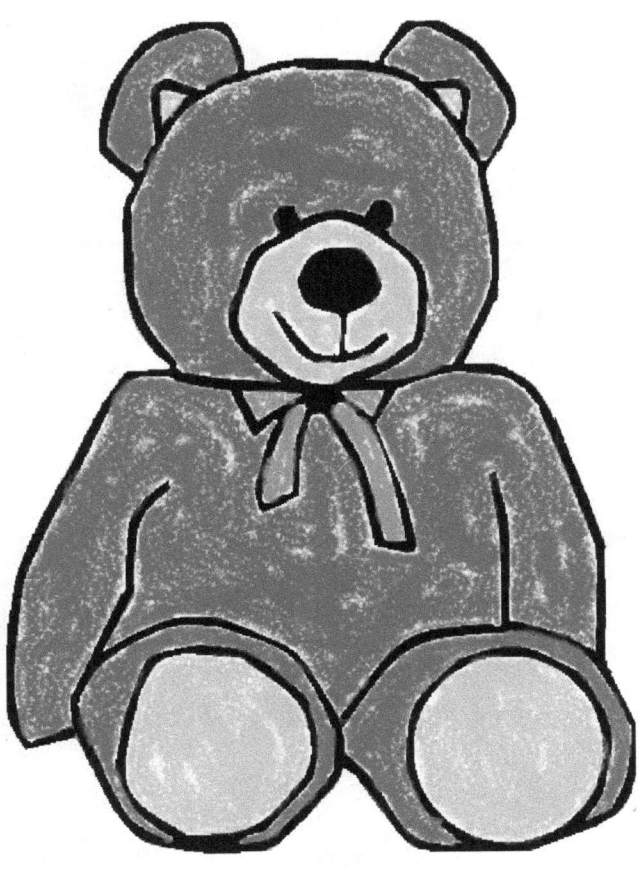

A coloring
book for a kid
with a premature
baby brother.

By S.E. Burr

I have a baby brother.

He is very, very small.

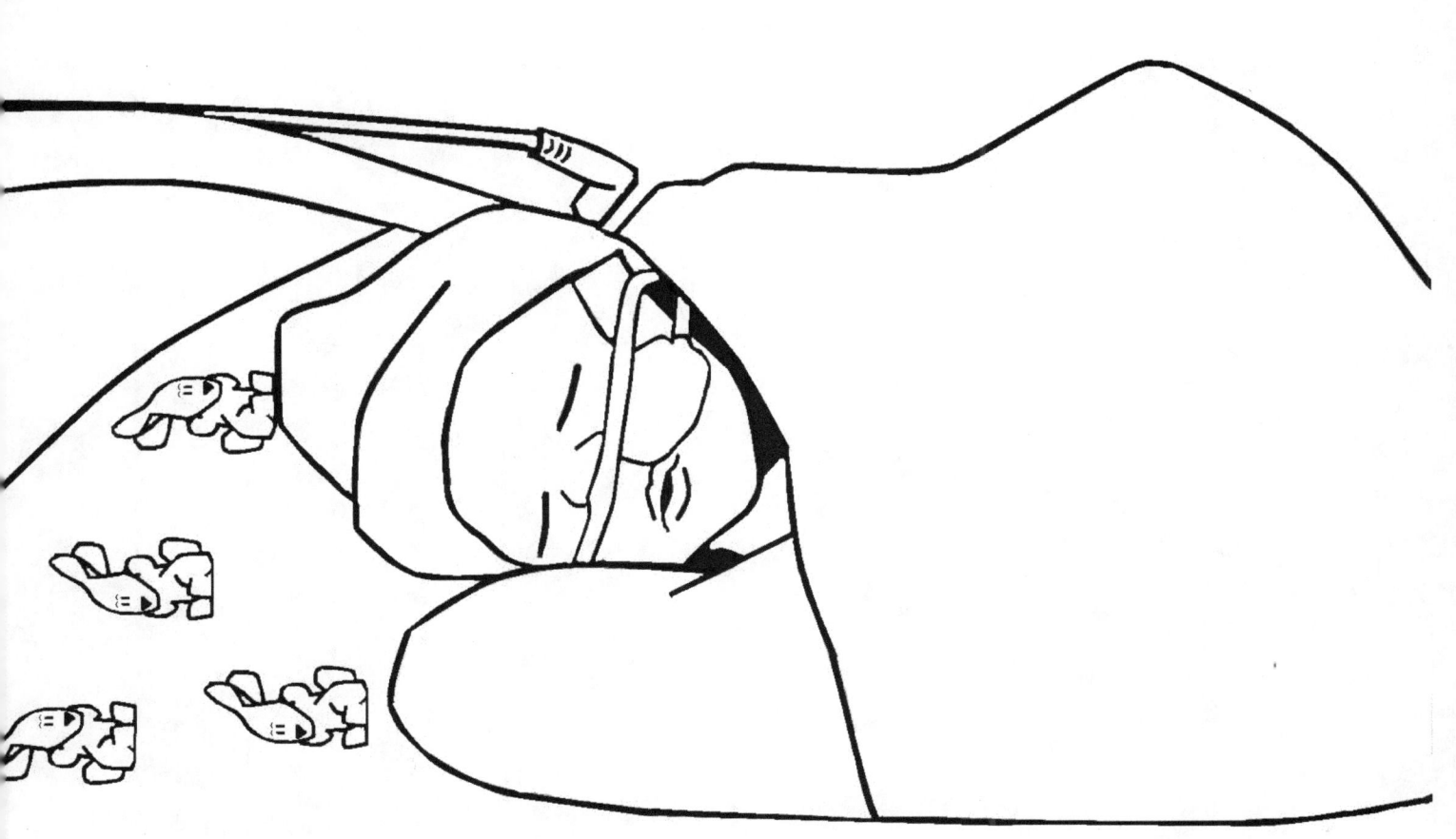

I am his older sibling.

I am big, and strong, and tall.

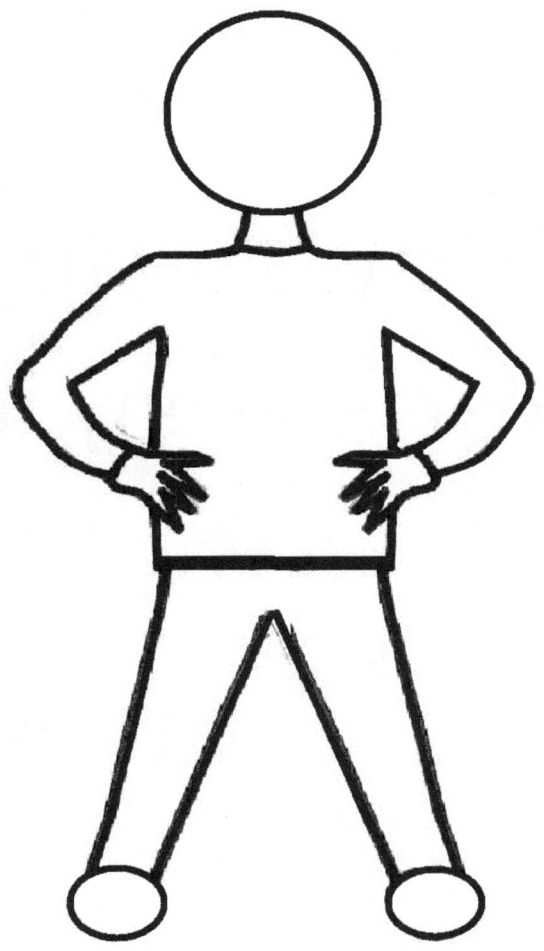

This is you! What does your hair look like? What color are your eyes? What kind of clothes do you like to wear? Draw yourself!

He has itty-bitty fingers
and teeny-weeny toes.

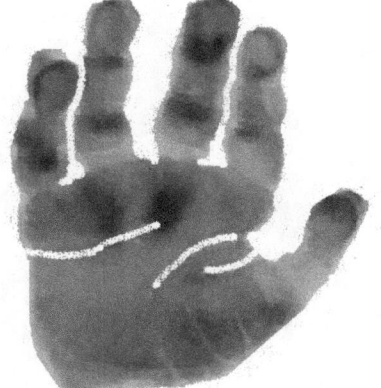
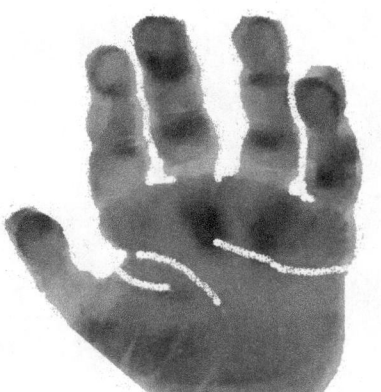

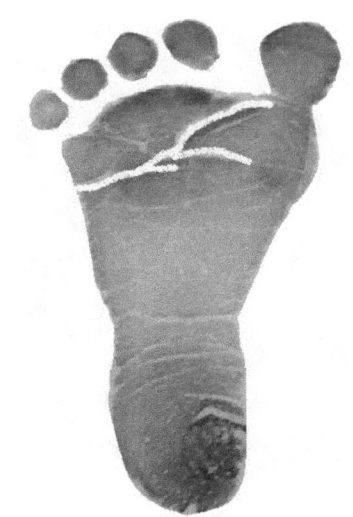
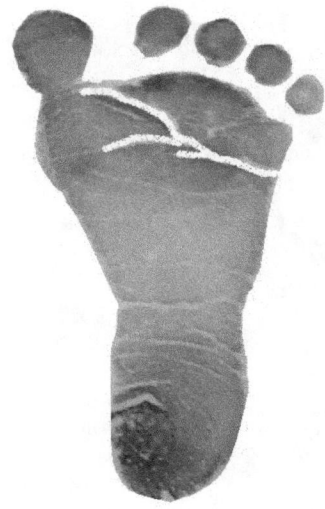

All of him is tiny,

from his feet up to his nose.

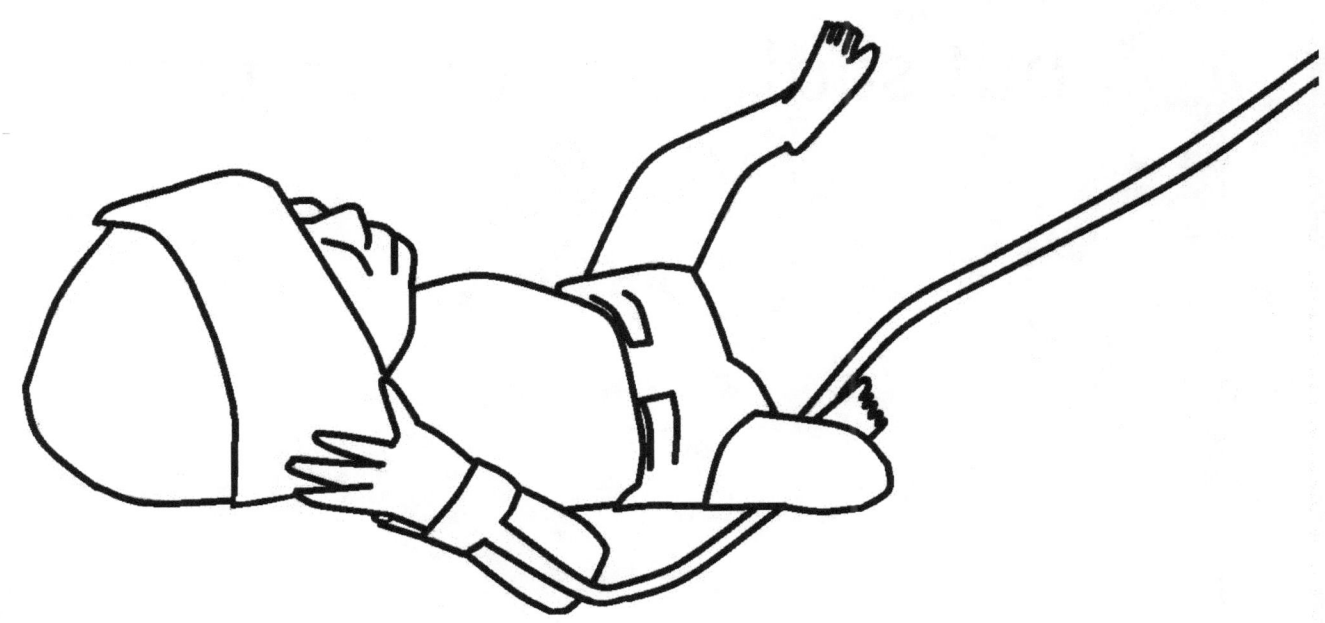

He was in my mommy's belly but sadly, he couldn't stay.

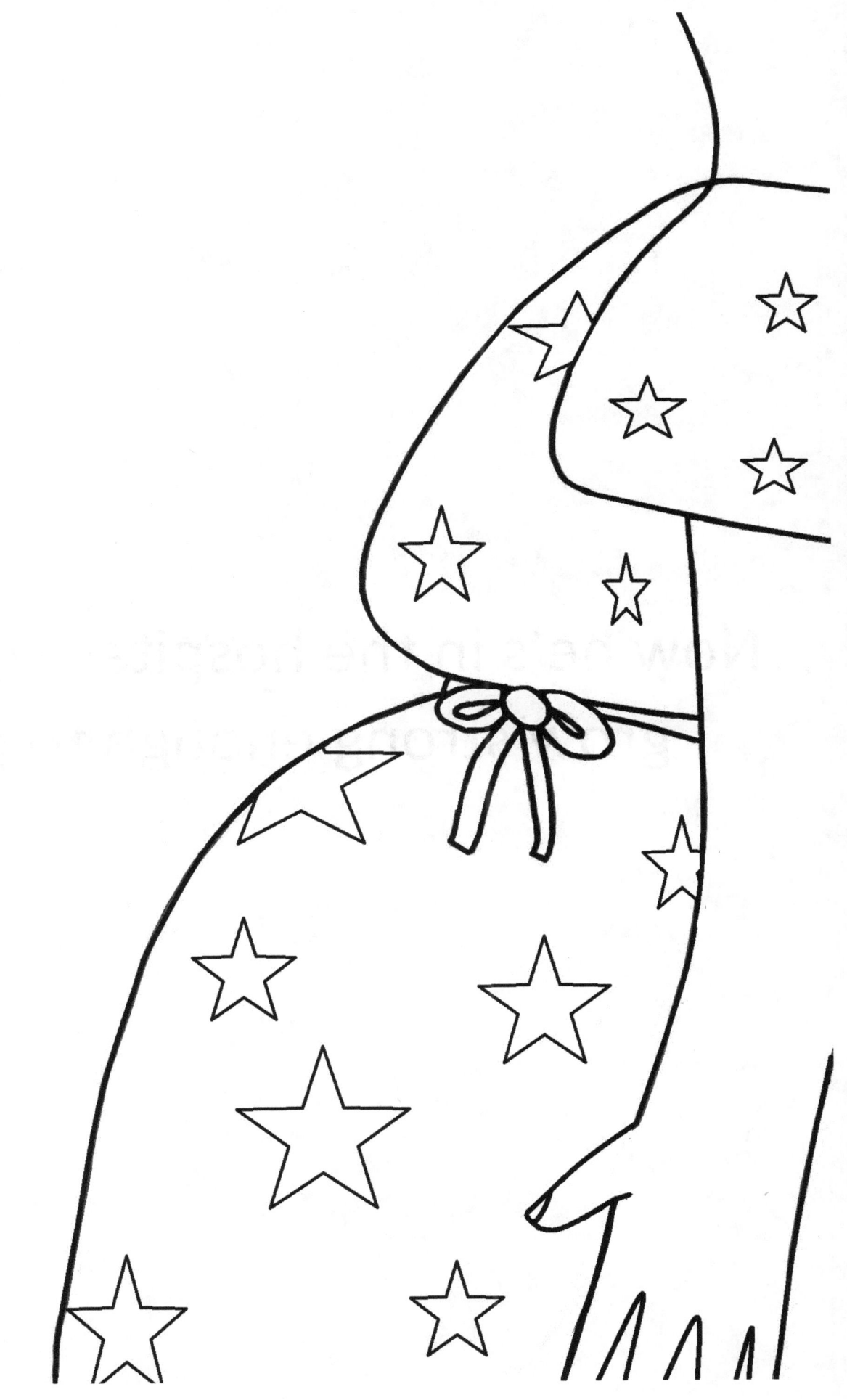

Now he's in the hospital, so he can grow strong enough to play.

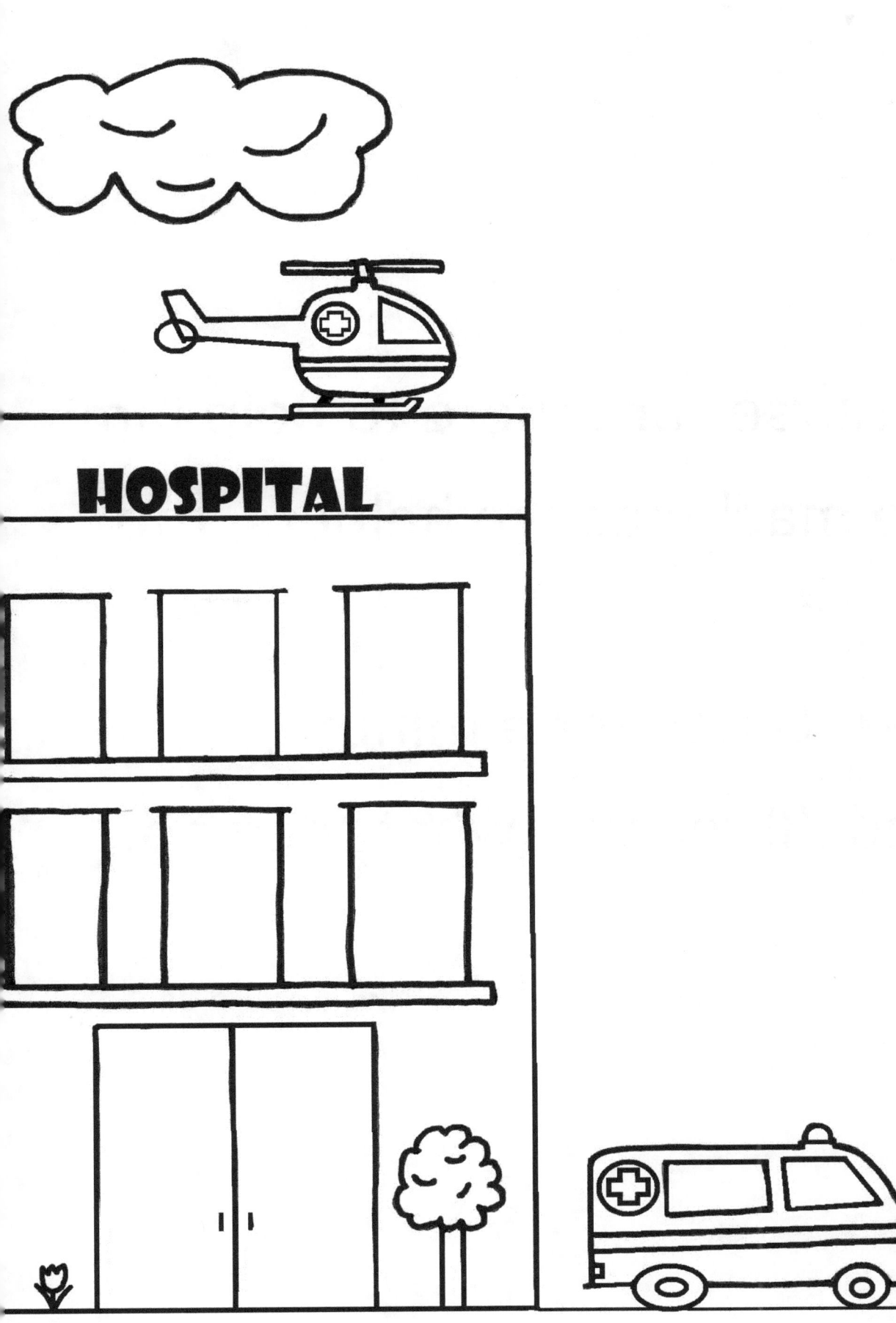

The nurses are there to help him.

The machines are helpers, too.

Listen for a minute,

and I'll tell you what they do.

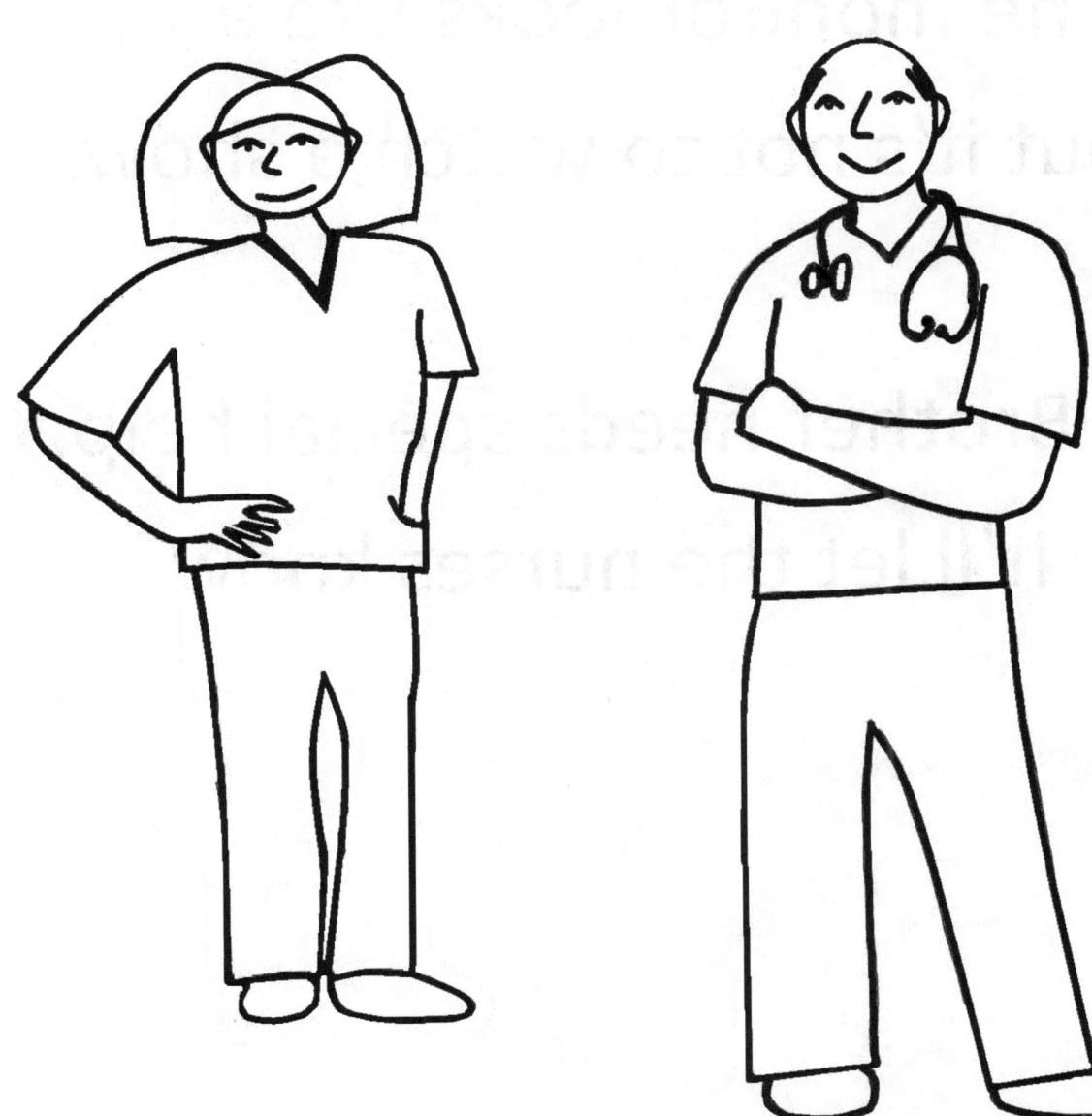

The monitor looks like a TV,
but it's not to watch a show.

If Brother needs special help,
it'll let the nurses know.

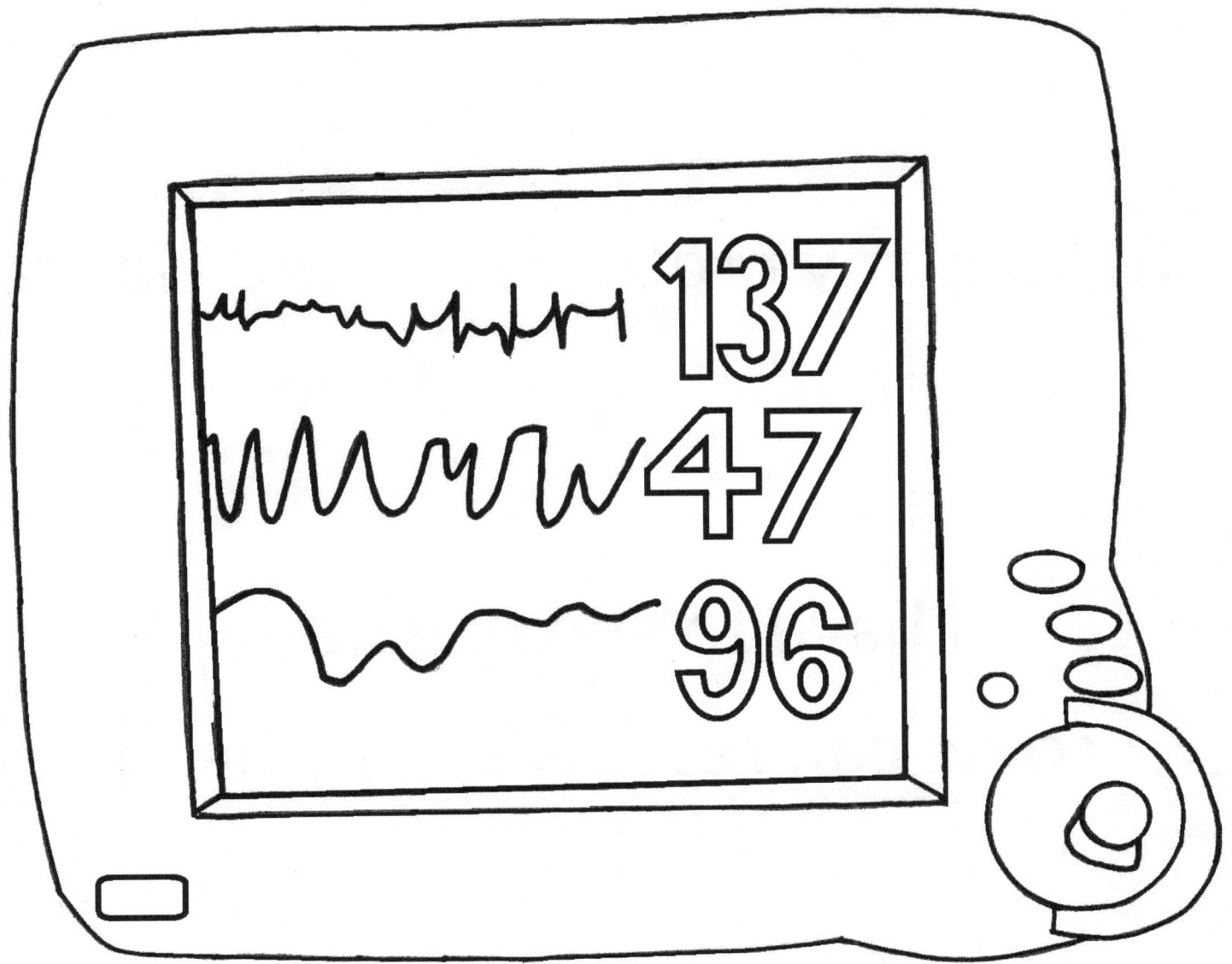

To keep my brother safe and warm,
he has a special bed.

I have to speak quietly
so he can rest his sleepy head.

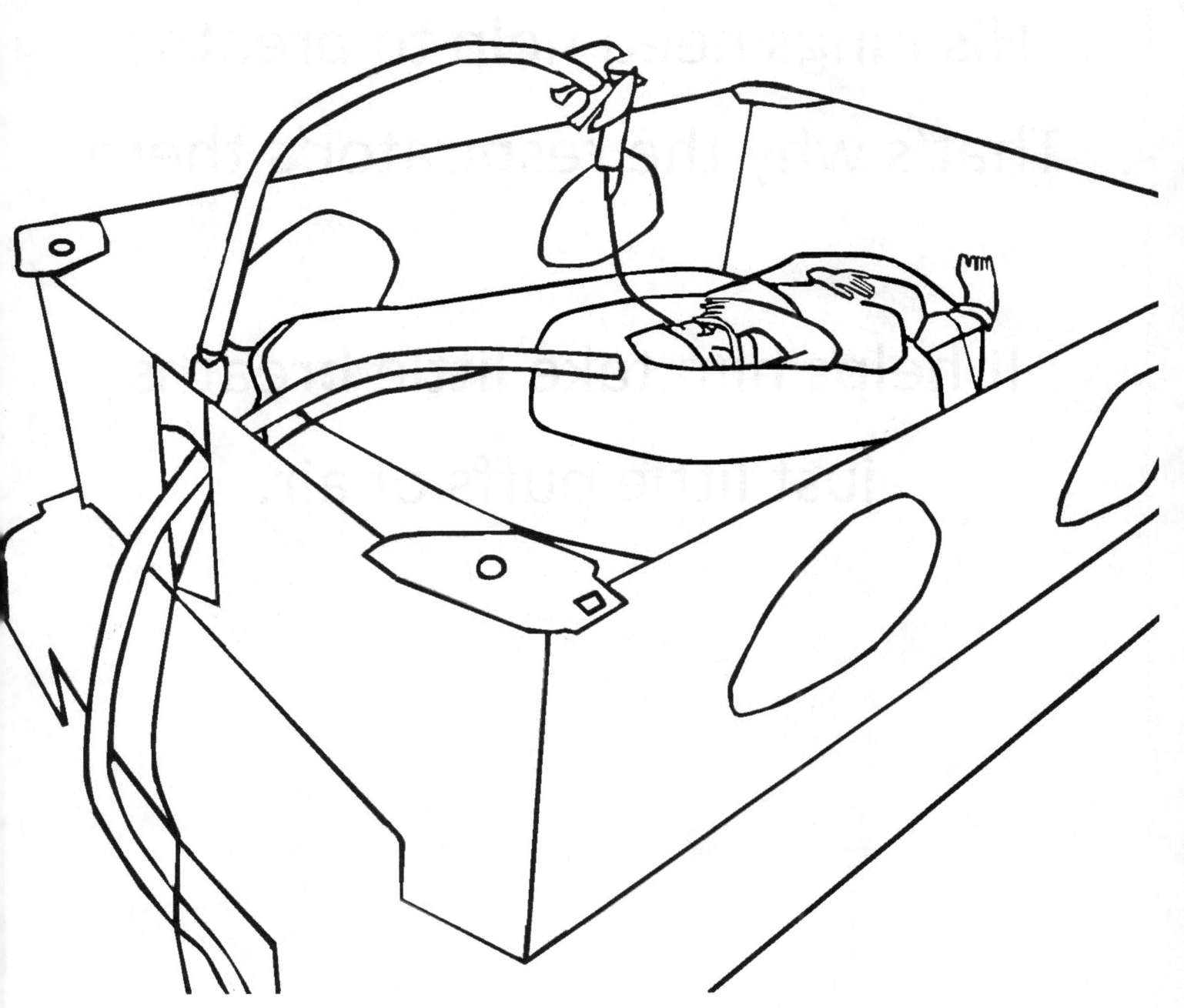

His lungs need help to breathe.
That's why the respirator's there.

It helps him take little breaths,
just little puffs of air.

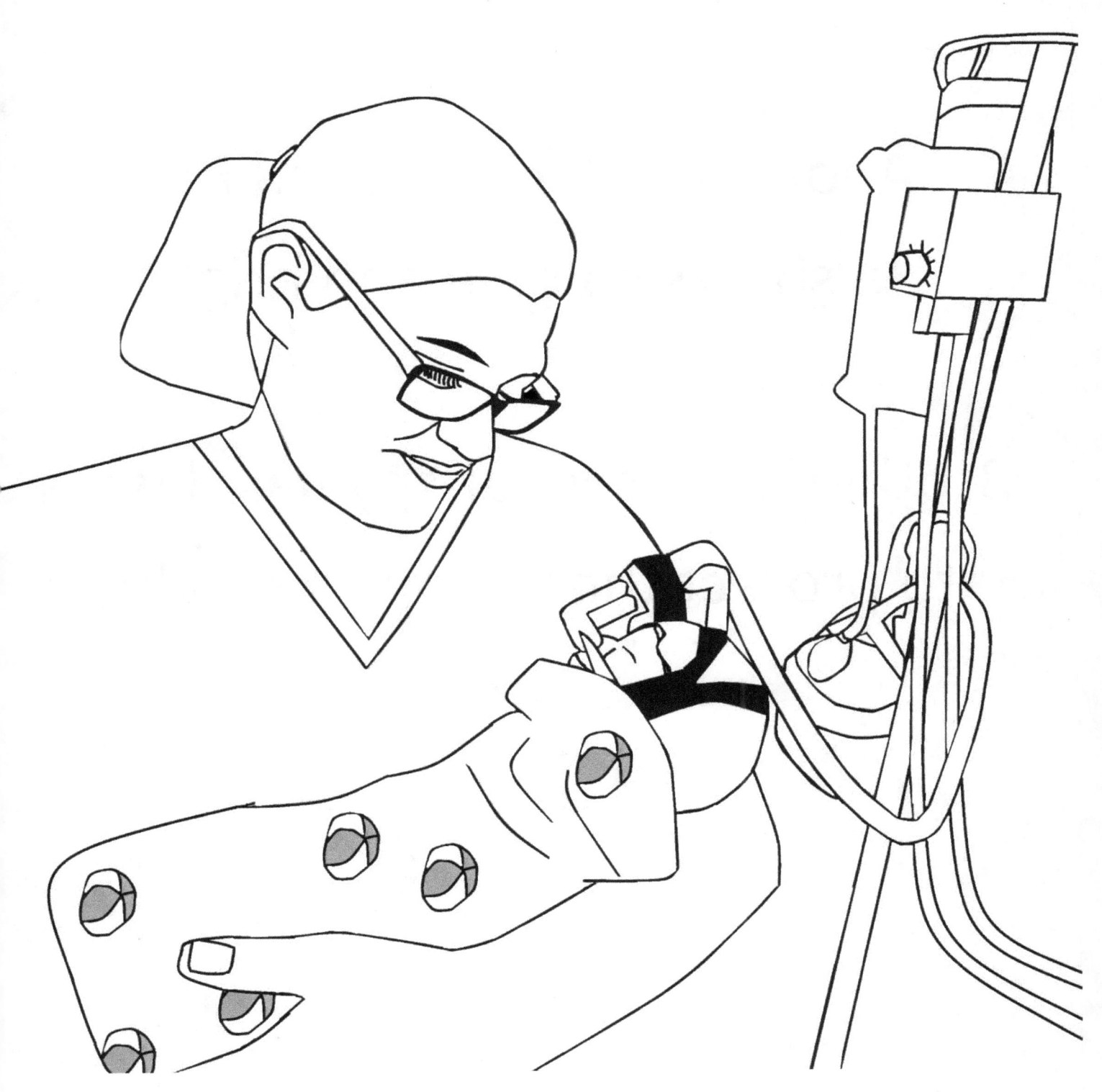

Another helper is called Bili.

He shines so blue and bright.

Brother's eyes wear special glasses
to protect them from the light.

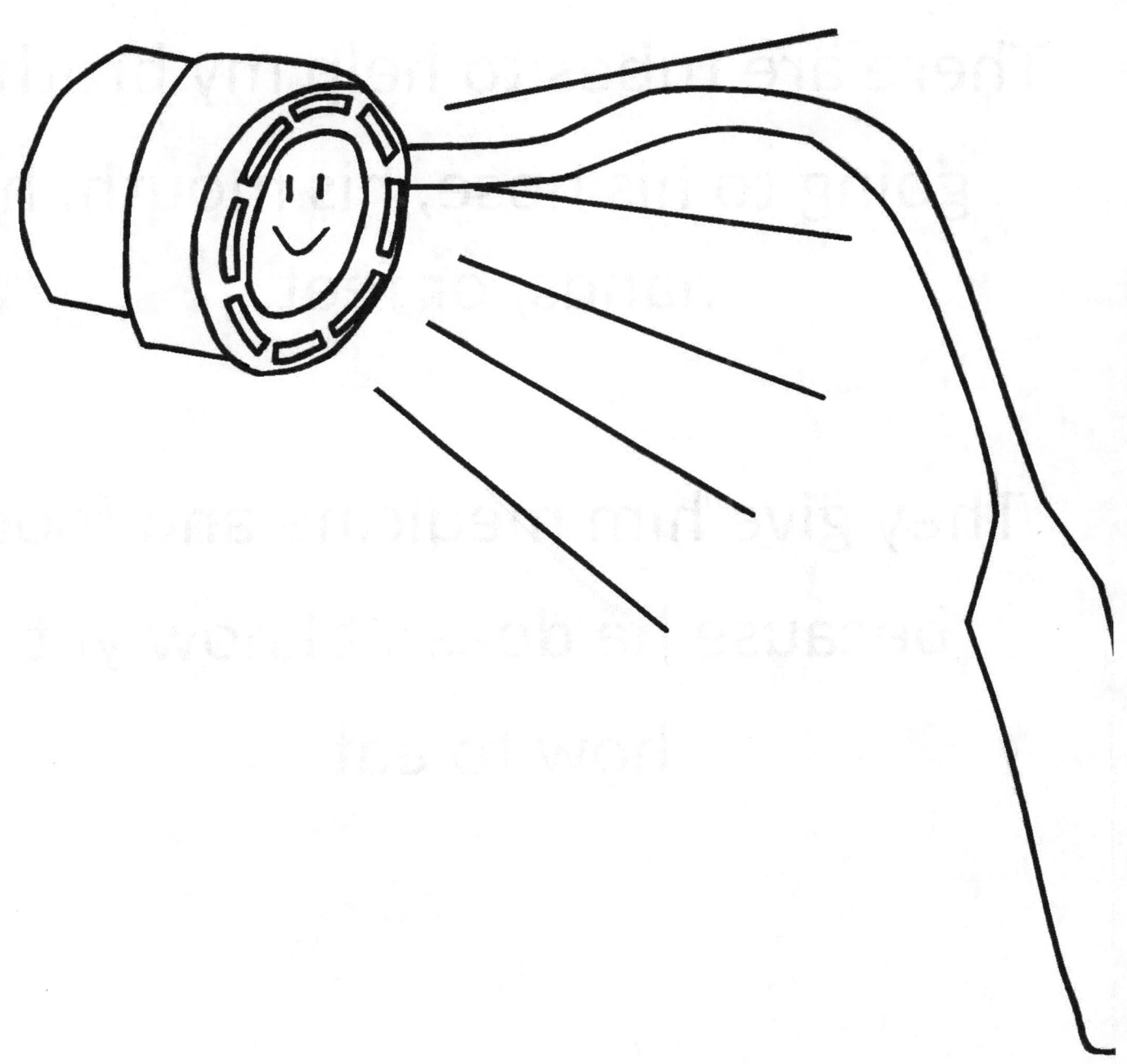

There are tubes to help my brother going to his nose, his mouth, his hands, or feet.

They give him medicine and food, because he doesn't know yet how to eat.

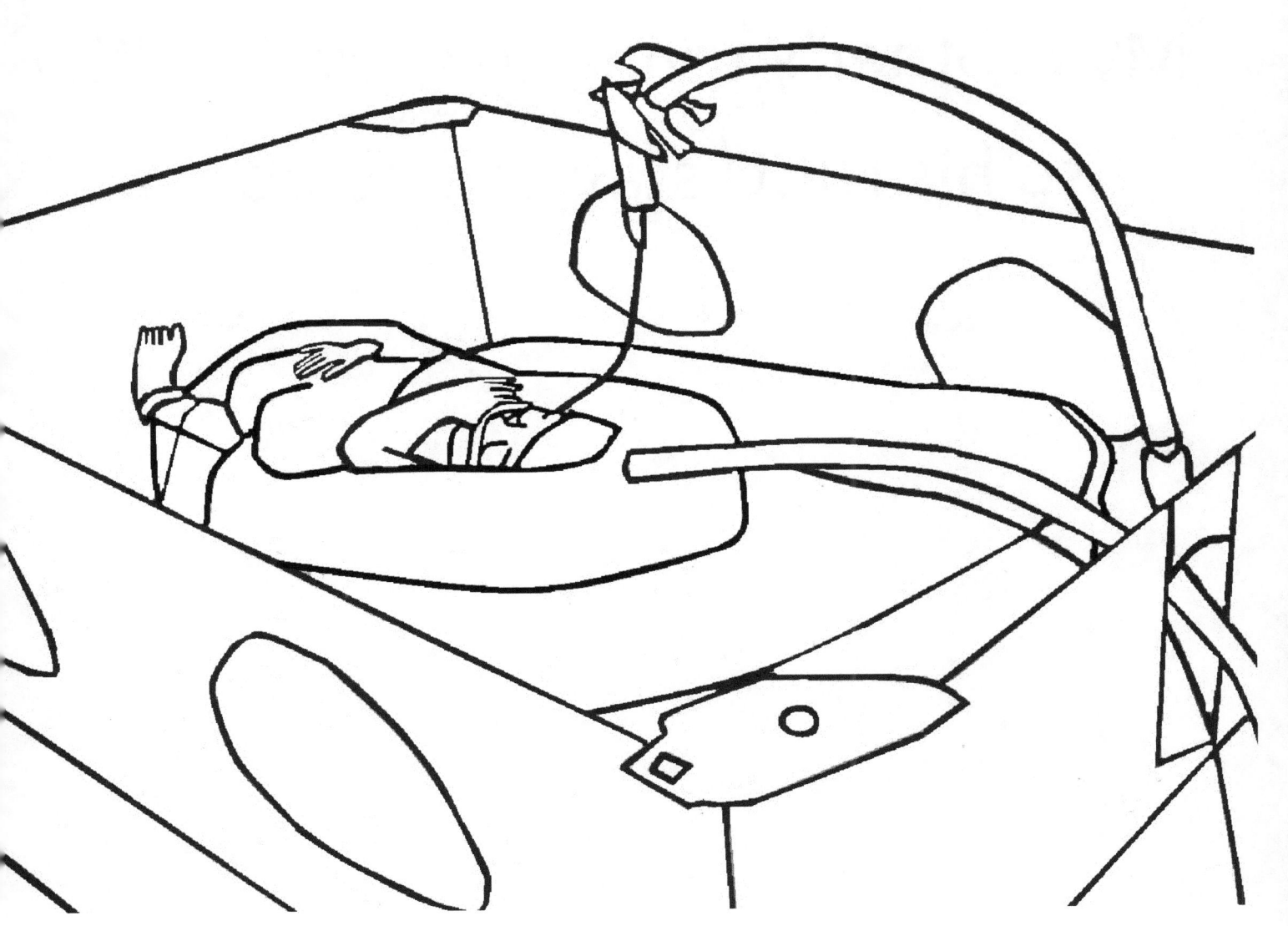

My brother's trying to grow healthy
so his NICU stay can be done.

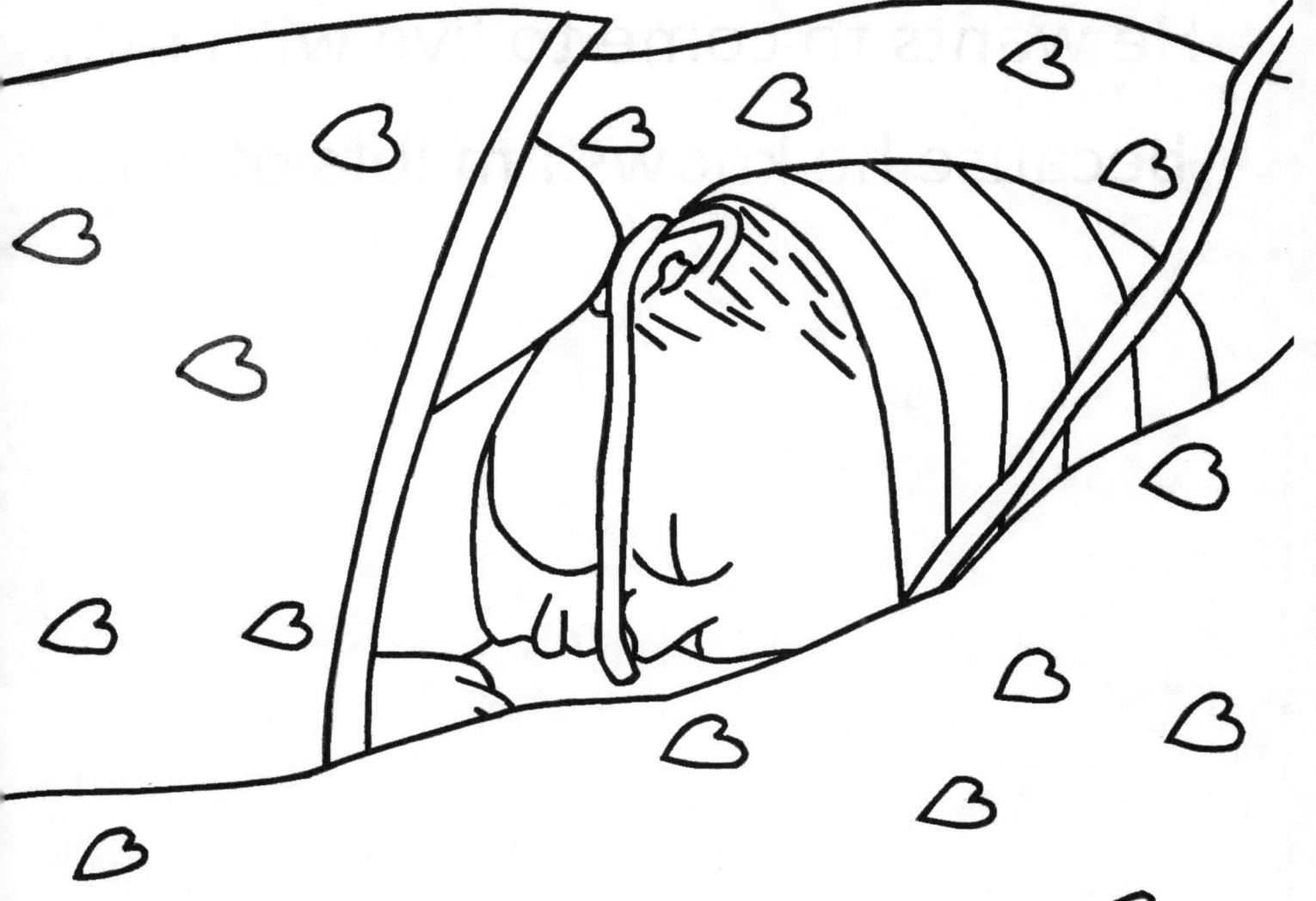

He wants to come to live with me, because he knows I'm lots of fun.

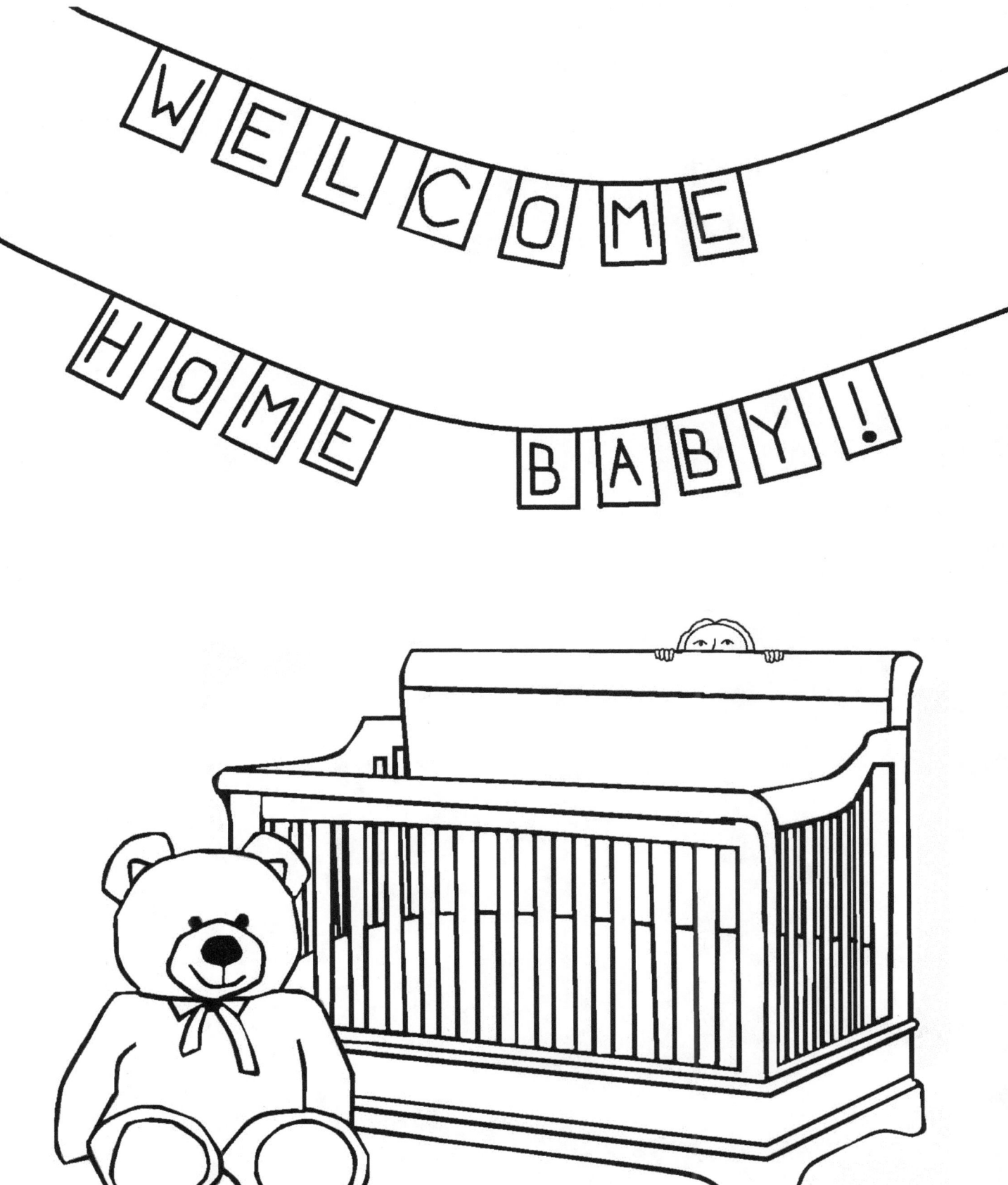

Printed in the USA
CPSIA information can be obtained
at www.ICGtesting.com
LVHW081158141223
766279LV00016B/657

9 781728 745459